# HELLO
## SOMEDAY

D1568096

WRITTEN BY KOBI YAMADA
& JOHN CHRISTIANSON

DESIGNED BY HEIDI DYER

# SOMEDAY IS HERE

YOU'VE ARRIVED AT THE CORNER OF "WHAT IF?" AND "WHY NOT?" IT'S THE PLACE WHERE YOU GET TO EXPLORE YOUR HOPES, DREAMS, AND ASPIRATIONS. SO MUCH OF LIFE HAS BEEN STRUCTURED AROUND OBLIGATIONS, RESPONSIBILITIES, AND TO-DO LISTS. BUT NOW YOU ARE TURNING THE PAGE TO A BRAND NEW CHAPTER. A CHAPTER THAT OPENS UP TO PASSIONS, POSSIBILITIES, AND CAN'T-WAIT-TO-DO LISTS.

For much of the entire history of the human race, the average life span was less than 30 years. There was no planning for retirement because there was no retirement. But with longer life spans, there is more time to think about and more ways to plan for the future. It's up to you to turn that something extra into something extraordinary.

One way to do this is to explore your interests and what you love about your life. Science shows that writing things down has a powerful and transformative effect on making them happen. It alters our thinking and ourselves in fundamental ways. This book is designed for you to do just that. You'll find questions, activities, and inspirations to get you started, and plenty of space for you to capture your thoughts and reflections along the way.

## HERE'S THE THING. THIS IS YOUR TIME.

If you want something but it doesn't exist, it's up to you to make it. Create the art you want to see, invent the product you want to use, write the book you want to read, make the dish you want to taste, sing the song you want to hear. It's your time to design the life you want to live.

# ...if you don't know where you're going, any road will take you there.

GEORGE HARRISON

As you begin your retirement journey, your level of financial readiness for the road ahead is likely top of mind. The reality is that money and financial subjects can create stress and anxiety, and this is completely normal. In fact, no matter how much financial preparation has been done, if any, everyone wants their retirement years to be filled with clarity, confidence, and peace of mind.

Just as the yellow line on a highway keeps you traveling in the right direction, the following financial checklist will help increase the odds of reaching your intended destination safely.

## GETTING THE BASICS DONE

I HAVE A BUDGET AND FINANCIAL PLAN.

MY WILL AND ESTATE PLAN ARE UP-TO-DATE.

I HAVE A VARIETY OF INVESTMENTS AND UNDERSTAND WHAT I OWN.

MY HEALTH INSURANCE AND LONG-TERM CARE NEEDS HAVE BEEN REVIEWED RECENTLY.

I KNOW WHEN I WILL START RECEIVING SOCIAL SECURITY AND PENSION PAYMENTS.

I HAVE A PROFESSIONAL TEAM (FINANCIAL ADVISOR, CPA, ATTORNEY, INSURANCE BROKER) TO GIVE ME ADVICE WHEN I NEED IT.

I HAVE IMPORTANT CONTACT INFORMATION ABOUT MY FINANCES AVAILABLE FOR CLOSE FAMILY AND TRUSTED FRIENDS THAT IS EASILY ACCESSIBLE.

## EXTRA CREDIT

BENEFICIARIES OF MY LIFE INSURANCE AND RETIREMENT ACCOUNTS ARE UP-TO-DATE.

MY INSURANCE POLICIES HAVE BEEN REVIEWED FOR PROPER COVERAGE AND LIMITS.

I HAVE REDUCED THE NUMBER OF INVESTMENTS AND BANK ACCOUNTS TO MAKE MY LIFE SIMPLER.

# LET YOUR HEART ILLUMINATE THE PATH BEFORE YOU.

After retiring, many people want to renew and refine their personal goals. "What do I do now?" is a common question as they find they have more to give. And they need to find new ways to focus their time and talents. For many, much of their identity and sense of purpose has been wrapped up in their work. And though it may seem illogical, extra time and fewer daily constraints can be challenging.

## DISCOVERING HOW YOU CAN MAKE YOUR UNIQUE CONTRIBUTION TO THE WORLD CAN ADD TREMENDOUS ENERGY TO YOUR LIFE.

*The following questions can help you examine your post-retirement journey:*

# WHO ARE YOU?

LIST YOUR TOP 3 CORE VALUES.

# WHAT ARE
# YOU GOOD AT?

LIST YOUR 3 BEST TALENTS OR COMPETENCIES.

WHAT ARE YOU EXCITED ABOUT?

WHAT WOULD BRING YOU THE MOST
PURPOSE AND MEANING?

LIST YOUR HIGHEST HOPE FOR
YOURSELF AND YOUR LIFE.

VISUALIZING A CLEAR PICTURE of something you want triggers the brain to subconsciously move toward that outcome. For example, golfers use a "pre-shot" routine and stand behind their ball to visualize their swing and the flight path of the ball before hitting their shot.

---

HOW WOULD IT FEEL TO HAVE A CLEAR PICTURE OF WHAT YOUR IDEAL FUTURE LOOKS LIKE? A NORTH STAR THAT INSPIRES YOUR DAILY ACTIONS?

*Here are some questions to help you to envision that future:*

# WHAT DOES SUCCESS MEAN TO YOU?

(PERSONALLY, PROFESSIONALLY, FINANCIALLY)

# WHAT DOES FIVE YEARS FROM NOW LOOK AND FEEL LIKE TO YOU?

# WHAT ABOUT TEN YEARS FROM NOW?

# WHAT ARE THE FORCES OR FEARS THAT ARE HOLDING YOU BACK?

# TODAY WANTS YOU TO COME OUT AND PLAY.

# It is important to remember that the beginning can be anywhere along the way.

UNKNOWN

How many times do we avoid starting something because we feel we need to be at an accomplished, master level right away?

When you start anything new, you will most likely be surrounded by coaches, teachers, or other people who probably have had the advantage of years of experience. We often compare our beginning abilities to those around us instead of having the patience to allow our skills to develop naturally over time.

WHAT IF YOU TOOK A NEW APPROACH?

_____

WHAT IF YOU LOOKED FORWARD TO
THE UNKNOWN AND THE POSSIBILITY
OF GROWTH?

_____

WHAT IF YOU EMBRACED BEING A BEGINNER
AND ENJOYED THE PROCESS AND FREEDOM
OF LEARNING WITHOUT EXPECTATION
OR JUDGMENT?

A MOTTO is a sentence or a turn of phrase that expresses a person's spirit, purpose, or guiding principle.

# WHAT'S YOUR LIFE MOTTO?

HERE ARE SOME EXAMPLES:

*Live a life you love.*

*Everything with intention.*

*Do it for the fun of it.*

*Imagine the impossible.*

*Be brave.*

# LIFE IS TOO SHORT TO...

# LIFE IS TOO SHORT NOT TO...

THERE IS A WORTHWHILE benefit to focusing
your time and energy on the things you can control,
instead of the things you can't. For example, you can
control (in varying degrees) your spending, investment costs, and taxes. On the other hand, you can't
control the direction of the stock or bond markets,
interest rates, or global economic events.

Controllable expenses can contribute positively to your
bottom line. Spending time stressing and worrying
about the uncontrollable influences just doesn't pay off.

The easiest controllable cost is your spending because
you alone set your lifestyle needs. If you don't know
what your total spending looks like, consider keeping
track of your spending for one month. By setting a budget
and reviewing your spending, it's common to find
unnecessary expenses and opportunities to simplify.

| CATEGORY | $ | PURPOSE OF EXPENSE |
|---|---|---|
| HOME AND UTILITIES | | |
| FOOD | | |
| DEBT | | |
| TRANSPORTATION | | |
| EDUCATION | | |
| SAVINGS | | |
| GIFTS AND CHARITY | | |
| TRAVEL | | |
| CLOTHING | | |
| PETS | | |
| ENTERTAINMENT | | |
| INSURANCE | | |
| HEALTH CARE | | |
| TAXES | | |
| PERSONAL AND MISC. | | |
| | | |

# WE'RE ALL STORIES IN THE END.

STEVEN MOFFAT

WHY ARE STORIES ABOUT US IMPORTANT?
THEY TRANSPORT US TO ANOTHER TIME,
HELP US TO LEARN ABOUT OUR PAST, AND
GUIDE US TOWARD OUR FUTURE. THEY ARE
A WAY WE CAN RELIVE OUR EXPERIENCES,
OUR LOVES, OUR ADVENTURES, OUR
DREAMS, AND OUR LIVES.

# GETTING TO KNOW YOU

We can be so involved with our day-to-day lives that we don't often reflect and reminisce on some of the most important things that have influenced and shaped who we are.

*Take time to interview yourself. Here are some questions to get you started:*

WHAT IS YOUR
PROUDEST MOMENT
SO FAR?

WHAT IS YOUR BEST
CHILDHOOD MEMORY?

WHAT DO YOU
LOVE MOST ABOUT
YOURSELF?

WHAT ALWAYS BRINGS
A SMILE TO YOUR FACE?

WHAT WOULD YOU LIKE
TO HAVE HAPPEN IN
YOUR LIFE THIS YEAR?

WHAT AREAS OF
GROWTH WOULD YOU
LIKE TO EXPERIENCE?

WHAT THINGS
WOULD YOU LIKE TO
STOP DOING?

WHERE WOULD YOU
LIKE TO GO?

# The things you are passionate about are not random, they are your calling.

FABIENNE FREDRICKSON

Passions are a road map to your
heart and soul. It's important
to listen to them, to follow them,
to see where they lead.

HOW WOULD YOU DESCRIBE WHAT YOU
WANT MOST IN LIFE?

_____

IF YOU HAD TO START SOMETHING TODAY,
AND IT WOULD BECOME YOUR LIFE'S
GREATEST WORK, WHAT WOULD IT BE?

_____

WHAT IS ONE CAUSE THAT IS WORTHY
OF YOUR TIME AND TALENTS?

_____

WHAT IS ONE CHANGE YOU WOULD LIKE
TO SEE HAPPEN IN YOUR LIFETIME?

_____

# INSPIRATION IS EVERYWHERE

How do you find inspiration? Is it a certain time of day or a feeling? Is it when you are with a particular person or at an especially meaningful place? Does it help to plan for it or does it find you at serendipitous times? Inspiration isn't something that can be forced, but it is something that can be welcomed.

WHAT IS AN OBJECT
THAT IS MOST
MEANINGFUL TO YOU?

WHAT IS A SONG THAT
ENERGIZES YOU AND
LIFTS YOUR SPIRITS?

WHAT IS A PLACE THAT
MAKES YOU FEEL MOST
COMFORTABLE?

WHAT IS A TASTE
THAT REMINDS YOU
OF HOME?

WHAT IS A SMELL
THAT RELAXES AND
CALMS YOU?

WHAT TIME OF DAY ARE
YOU MOST CREATIVE?

WHEN DO YOU FEEL
MOST CONNECTED
AND LOVED?

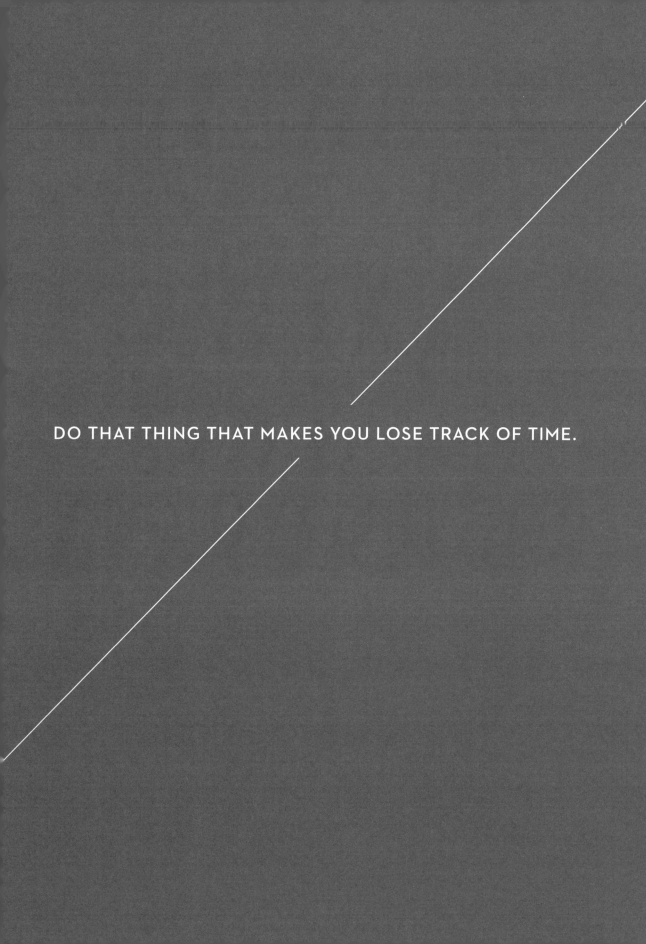

DO THAT THING THAT MAKES YOU LOSE TRACK OF TIME.

The word *meraki* is a word that modern Greeks often use to describe what happens when you leave a piece of yourself, your soul, creativity, or love, in your work. Maybe it's a song, or a piece of pottery, or a painting? Or perhaps it's a spread-sheet, a beautiful algorithm, or a recipe. When you love doing something, anything, so much that you put something of yourself into it...

*that is meraki.*

# WHERE DOES MERAKI EXIST FOR YOU?

# Do you believe that risk goes down as you get older?

Most people view this question primarily as a financial one—by looking for ways to decrease their investment risk as they age. But we can become inflexible in other ways, too. Flexibility, in every area of your life, is the key to living well.

Flexing these "risk muscles" can mean being willing to take a chance. Many of the best outcomes in life come from being willing to risk something. You may not be willing to risk your money, but what about risking your time, your experience, your passion, your connections, and your imagination for something important to you? Perhaps those muscles can be used to nurture a new friendship, start a community garden, mentor young business leaders, coach a youth sports team, teach a class at the high school, or volunteer at the local food shelter.

WHY NOT INCREASE YOUR RISK
TOLERANCE FOR SOMETHING
YOU LOVE NOW THAT YOU HAVE
MORE TIME AND OPPORTUNITY
TO BRANCH OUT, TRY SOMETHING
NEW, AND MAKE A DIFFERENCE?

# Indeed, what is there that does not appear marvelous when it comes to our knowledge for the first time?

PLINY THE ELDER

WHEN WAS THE LAST TIME you did something for the first time?
One of the greatest feelings is experiencing something brand
new. When something is new to us, our senses are awake and we
come alive. There is an added luster and brightness; we feel like
we are really experiencing and living life. Do you remember your
first kiss? The first time you put your toes in the ocean? The first
time you boarded an airplane? Firsts are exhilarating and exciting
times that make us feel alive.

LIST 3 EXPERIENCES
YOU WANT BUT
HAVEN'T HAD YET.

SOME PEOPLE make your laugh a little louder, your smile a little brighter, your heart a little bigger, and your life a little better. They seem to have a light all their own. And the longer you live, the more you realize who really matters, who never did, and who always will. The people you look up to say a lot about you and your values.

LIST 5 PEOPLE YOU ADMIRE MOST IN THE WORLD
*and what you admire about them.*

BACK IN 2002, educator Nínive Clements Calegari and author Dave Eggers were looking for a way to support overburdened teachers and to connect talented working adults with students who could use their help. They wanted to open a free tutoring center. They settled on a building in the Mission District of San Francisco at 826 Valencia Street that housed a weight-training gym before closing down for a number of years. The location was perfect, but there was a bit of a hiccup: the city government effectively told them, "That's nice that you want to open a free tutoring center, but that building is zoned for retail, so you're going to have to sell something." Unsure of how to proceed—certainly they shouldn't charge for tutoring—the solution emerged during a building renovation session. The building needed a lot of T.L.C., and stripping out the old tiles revealed beautiful, old, whitewashed rafters that had just the right amount of wear to look rustic. So perfectly rustic, in fact, that somebody said, "It feels like you're inside an old ship."

AND SO, A CRAZY IDEA WAS BORN:

The 826 Valencia Pirate Supply Store, where anyone can come purchase peg legs, eye patches, compasses, and all other various and sundry provisions. Incredibly, the store has proven to be a real asset for the center, with all of its proceeds used to help fund the organization's operations. Furthermore, it firmly established 826 as a space that is imaginative, special, and altogether magical.

The writing lab was built behind the store and was designed to be a place where kids would want to spend time. Word spread quickly, and soon every chair was filled. Since opening, 826 Valencia has helped thousands of students work on their writing with an army of trained volunteer tutors.

THINK OF A POTENTIAL PROBLEM OR OPPORTUNITY YOU'D LIKE TO TACKLE—IN YOUR COMMUNITY, YOUR CITY, OR EVEN YOUR OWN HOME. HOW COULD YOU REINVENT YOURSELF TO MAKE IT HAPPEN?

# By doing what you love, you inspire and awaken the hearts of others.

UNKNOWN

# WHAT MAKES YOU SMILE?

*Circle the ones that apply to you and fill in a few of your own.*

LIFE'S LITTLE PLEASURES ARE
EVERYWHERE AND ALL AROUND US.
THEY ARE JUST WAITING FOR US
TO NOTICE AND APPRECIATE THEM.

ICE CREAM NICE PEOPLE UNEXPECTED KINDNESS
ACTS OF GENEROSITY ELBOW ROOM PUPPIES
FAMILY DINNERS LONG HUGS GOOD MANNERS
DANCING WARM COOKIES A GOOD BOOK
FRESHLY CUT FLOWERS SHOES ON THE PORCH
FREE TIME CHILDREN LAUGHING FIREFLIES
SHARING STORIES A HANDWRITTEN NOTE
A JOB WELL DONE OPEN MINDS CARD GAMES
A COMPASSIONATE GESTURE BIG HEARTS
DEEP BELLY LAUGHS WATCHING THE CLOUDS
FARMERS' MARKETS A SEVENTH-INNING STRETCH
A NICE BOTTLE OF WINE SINGING OFF-KEY
THE OPEN ROAD NATURE WALKS STARRY NIGHTS
GOOD DEALS A MORNING CUP OF COFFEE
HOLDING HANDS A COZY FIRE...

_____

_____

_____

# intention

*[in-ten-shuhn] noun*

---

1  An act or instance of determining mentally upon some action or result.

2  Purpose or attitude toward the effect of one's actions or conduct.

3  A necessary tool for living a life on purpose.

# I WILL...

share my talents

make new mistakes

take a class

IF YOU HAVEN'T FOUND IT YET, KEEP LOOKING.

One glance at a book and you hear the voice of another person, perhaps someone dead for 1,000 years. To read is to voyage through time.

An adventure awaits, all you have to do is take it... It's waiting for you on your bookshelf or at your local library. Now that you have more time, what are the things you are interested in or curious about? What are the places you want to discover? Who are the people you want to know better? Great stories, faraway lands, grand adventures, future worlds, and historical insights are always at your fingertips. You just have to open a book. Maybe you want to revisit an old favorite of yours? Or dive into a current best seller? The options are endless, and they are all waiting for you.

LIST 3 OF YOUR
FAVORITE BOOKS
OF ALL TIME.

LIST 3 BOOKS
YOU REALLY WANT
TO READ.

# IF I HAD TO LIVE MY LIFE OVER AGAIN, I WOULD HAVE SPENT MORE TIME ON...

# IF I HAD TO LIVE MY LIFE OVER AGAIN, I WOULD HAVE SPENT LESS TIME ON...

Every morning you
have two choices:
continue to sleep with
your dreams, or wake
up and chase them.

UNKNOWN

I HOPE THAT IN THIS YEAR TO COME, YOU MAKE MISTAKES.

Because if you are making mistakes, then you are making new things, trying new things, learning, living, pushing yourself, changing yourself, changing your world. You're doing things you've never done before, and more importantly, you're Doing Something.

So that's my wish for you, and all of us, and my wish for myself. Make New Mistakes. Make glorious, amazing mistakes. Make mistakes nobody's ever made before. Don't freeze, don't stop, don't worry that it isn't good enough, or it isn't perfect, whatever it is: art, or love, or work or family or life.

Whatever it is you're scared of doing, Do it.

Make your mistakes, next year and forever.

Neil Gaiman

# WE DO NOT REMEMBER DAYS, WE REMEMBER MOMENTS.

CESARE PAVESE

WHAT A LIFE you've lived so far. Take some time to gather photos that make you feel happy—that remind you of the experiences, joys, loves, and laughter. Also gather pages from favorite books, handwritten letters you received, favorite words, thoughts, or quotations. Get an old picture frame from a vintage store or garage sale or a brand new one from a frame shop. Remove the glass and mount your treasures. Add as many or as few photos as you want. The important part is that it should make you feel good, and bring a smile to your face, just by looking at it. Spend a few minutes each day to reminisce, to study the details, to remember the stories and the emotions of why you chose each of them.

# If you could ask your great-great-grandparents anything, what would it be?

If you could talk to your
great-great-grandchildren,
what would you tell them?

# WHEN YOUR HEART SPEAKS, TAKE GOOD NOTES.

JUDITH EXNER

The world needs what you've got. There are countless worthy causes that need your time, talent, and resources. It only takes one person to make a difference, and that person can be you.

---

## WHAT ARE YOU INTERESTED/EXCITED/ CURIOUS/PASSIONATE ABOUT?

*Check all that apply or the one that means the most to you:*

| | | |
|---|---|---|
| | | EQUALITY |
| | | ENDING FAMINE AND POVERTY |
| | | SPORTS |
| | | ANIMAL WELFARE |
| | | FAMILY |
| | | YOUTH |
| | | CREATIVITY |
| | | ENVIRONMENTAL ISSUES |
| | | ARTS |
| | | SOCIAL CAUSES |
| | | CULTURE |
| | | TV/FILM/ENTERTAINMENT |
| | | LITERACY |
| | | HEALTH AND FITNESS |
| | | NUTRITION |
| | | OTHER: |

# What does it mean to be lucky?

HAVE YOU EVER NOTICED that some people just seem to be lucky in life? It's as if there is some magical force helping to make things go their way. Did you ever wonder how they do it? Do you ever wish you were a bit luckier? Well, it turns out, luck isn't just a matter of luck, it's actually something you can influence. The main difference between lucky people and unlucky people is their attitude and orientation to whatever is happening.

Lucky people tend to see setbacks as temporary obstacles to overcome and embrace fortuitous events with gratitude and appreciation. On the other hand, unlucky people see setbacks as confirmation that life is hard— and when things actually go their way, they minimize those occurrences and fear that something bad is just around the corner.

According to research by psychologist Richard Wiseman, there are ways to *learn* to be luckier. Feeling lucky is much less a special power you are born with and more of a habit you can develop. For starters, embrace optimism, try to see the bright side of challenging events, be open to new experiences, trust your gut, expect good things to happen, and maximize serendipitous opportunities.

SO WHETHER YOU THINK YOU ARE LUCKY OR NOT, YOU'RE PROBABLY RIGHT.

One day you will wake up and there won't be any more time to do the things you've always wanted.

# DO IT NOW.

PAULO COELHO

# Today is a perfect day for a perfect day.

## HOW WOULD YOU DESCRIBE
## YOUR PERFECT DAY?

HOW DOES IT START? WHERE ARE YOU?
WHAT DO YOU SEE? WHAT ARE YOU
DOING? WHO ARE YOU WITH? HOW DOES
IT FEEL? HOW DOES IT END?

A GROUP OF STUDENTS was asked to list what they thought were the current Seven Wonders of the World. Though there were some disagreements, the following received the most votes:

1. EGYPT'S GREAT PYRAMIDS
2. TAJ MAHAL
3. GRAND CANYON
4. PANAMA CANAL
5. EMPIRE STATE BUILDING
6. ST. PETER'S BASILICA
7. CHINA'S GREAT WALL

While gathering the votes, the teacher noted that one student had not finished her paper yet. So she asked the girl if she was having trouble with her list. The girl replied, "Yes, a little. I couldn't quite make up my mind because there are so many." The teacher said, "Well, tell us what you have, and maybe we can help." The girl hesitated, then read, "I think the Seven Wonders of the World are:

1. TO SEE
2. TO HEAR
3. TO TOUCH
4. TO TASTE
5. TO FEEL
6. TO LAUGH
7. AND TO LOVE."

*The room was so quiet you could have heard a pin drop.*

ORIGINALLY TOLD BY JOY GARRISON WASSON, AN ENGLISH TEACHER IN MUNCIE, INDIANA, FOR MORE THAN 30 YEARS.

# What simple, ordinary, everyday "wonders" do you overlook or take for granted?

...cultivate the habit of being grateful for every good thing that comes to you; and to give thanks continuously. And because all things have contributed to your advancement, you should include all things in your gratitude.

WALLACE WATTLES

Today, pick out a personalized piece of stationery
or a greeting card that feels right and pen a note
to someone who has made a difference in your life.
It could be a past mentor, a parent, a child, an old
friend, someone you worked with, or maybe someone
who believed in you before you believed in yourself.

_____

*A handwritten note from you, out of the blue,*
*will mean the world to them.*

_____

SOCIAL MEDIA can be a great way to feel connected, learn about the world, and share your interests. People of multiple generations are realizing that by going to social media, where their family members are going, it becomes easier to link up and keep up with what is going on in the lives of their loved ones. It also makes for more frequent and comfortable conversations, helping you all to feel closer as a family.

*Why do you choose social media?*

I FEEL MORE CONNECTED.

I FEEL A SENSE OF COMMUNITY.

IT KEEPS ME UP-TO-DATE ON THE WORLD.

I CAN SHARE MY INTERESTS.

I CAN SHARE PHOTOS AND VIDEOS.

IT'S FUN.

I CAN FIND NEW FRIENDS.

I CAN REDISCOVER OLD FRIENDS.

I'M INSPIRED BY OTHERS.

IT GIVES ME SOMETHING TO DO.

OTHER:

You have lived a rich and fulfilling life so far. A life that matters in so many ways. A life filled with moments and memories of laughter, learning, and living. A life with connections to people who have shaped you, cared for you, and loved you.

If you were to look back over your life, what would you want others to know about what is most meaningful to you?

IN MY LIFE, I ACHIEVED:

_____
_____
_____

I WAS LOVED BY:

_____
_____
_____

MOST FUN I EVER HAD:

_____
_____
_____

IMPORTANT PEOPLE IN MY LIFE WERE:

_____
_____
_____

I OWE A LOT TO:

_____
_____
_____

BEST ADVICE I RECEIVED:

_____
_____
_____

LESSONS I LEARNED:

_____
_____
_____

I WAS PASSIONATE ABOUT:

_____
_____
_____

I MADE A DIFFERENCE BY:

_____
_____
_____

I BELIEVED IN:

_____
_____
_____

I AM MOST GRATEFUL FOR:

_____
_____
_____

HAPPINESS TO ME IS:

_____
_____
_____

P.S.

_____
_____
_____
_____
_____

...I LOOK FORWARD TO ALL THAT I
CAN CONTRIBUTE TO THIS WORLD
BECAUSE OF MY AGE AND LIFE
EXPERIENCE IN A WAY THAT WOULD
HAVE BEEN IMPOSSIBLE AT HALF MY
AGE. I'M COOL WITH THAT.

NEIL DEGRASSE TYSON

AGE 57, ASTROPHYSICIST, AUTHOR,
SCIENCE SUPERSTAR, AND RECIPIENT
OF THE NATIONAL ACADEMY OF
SCIENCES' MOST PRESTIGIOUS AWARD
ON BEING ASKED IF HE WAS AFRAID
OF GETTING OLDER.

# HAVE THE TIME OF YOUR LIFE.

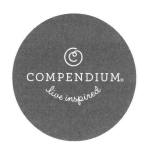

WITH SPECIAL THANKS TO THE ENTIRE COMPENDIUM FAMILY.

CREDITS:
Written by: Kobi Yamada
& John Christianson
Designed by: Heidi Dyer
Edited by: Amelia Riedler

ABOUT JOHN CHRISTIANSON, CFA
John is the founder and CEO of Highland Private Wealth
Management, Inc., a boutique financial advisory firm
that guides and stewards the wealth and aspirations
of business leaders and their families. John specializes
in coaching wealth creators who want a thoughtful
approach to integrating their life and money.
He calls it Living Fully™.

ISBN: 978-1-938298-96-7